Work out in 10 minutes.
Simple, Effective Exercises for Seniors to enhance a healthy living

By

Marc B. Wagner

Introduction

At the point when you age, your body changes, and it tends to be difficult to keep up
with the request of being a solid senior. In any case, this doesn't

mean there's no desire for keeping up with or working on your wellbeing
as you age. Contingent upon how old you are and how truly
dynamic you were in your more youthful years, a great many activities
are accessible to assist with keeping up with your wellness level and moving along
strength, power, and equilibrium. One thing that numerous seniors frequently
neglect is their eating regimen while settling on acclimations to food decisions
(for example, changing from vehicle to strolling, or strolling to trekking), work out (for example moving from the lounge chair to a customary work-out daily practice),
also, other way-of-life decisions (for example stopping smoking, getting more
rest) it's not difficult to disregard keeping a solid eating regimen that is
loaded with nutrients and supplements that can help your body
capability better as you age.
Practice is a significant piece of a general way of life change for seniors as it assists them with keeping up with the equilibrium, strength, and portability of maturing. Activities can likewise:
expansion to the medical advantages of activity, you might encounter a lift in your fearlessness, temperament, and energy levels.
Working out might in fact assist with alleviating pressure and uneasiness.
Numerous sorts of activities should be possible to assist with working on your actual well-being as you age. The

activity you pick relies upon your ongoing wellness level and objective. For instance, assuming strolling is

enough to get your pulse up as a component of an oxygen-consuming exercise,

you ought to do that. Then again, you may

need to attempt strength preparation assuming that you really want to work on your

strength.

Nearly everybody knows about cardio activities like running,

bicycling, and strolling. Vigorous activities get the pulse up to

where it's buckling down sufficiently so that oxygen is being

utilized productively by the muscles. Anaerobic activity is unique

from vigorous practice in that anaerobic exercises use oxygen at a

high rate yet are not effective enough for the muscles to ideally work. The vigorous activity utilizes oxygen the entire day, consistently, and for significant stretches. This exercise keeps a sound

heart and helps fabricate solid bones since it keeps your muscles solid and adaptable. Instances of vigorous activities are strolling, running, and trekking.

Opposition preparation helps tone muscles. It can help get to the next level

of muscle strength and power. Instances of opposition practices incorporate power lifting and body weight activities, for example, push-ups and squats. Obstruction preparation is an extraordinary method for keeping up with your solidarity level as you age since it helps develop your muscles. As we become older, our muscles become more vulnerable, so we

should keep major areas of strength for them by doing strength-preparing practices consistently.

Extending is another activity that further develops adaptability and equilibrium, which diminishes the possibility of falling and breaking a bone. Extending likewise helps the scope of movement in your joints.

Adaptability can assist you with keeping away from wounds and recuperating from specific wounds that might have happened due to falling.

Adaptability practices incorporate extending and strength preparing works out. Strength preparing practices are intended to develop the fortitude in your muscles, which helps support solid connective tissue (like ligament and ligaments) as well as assist you with keeping a sound weight. How frequently you want to stretch will rely upon your age, general well-being, wellness level, active work levels, climate, and different variables. A typical type of extending is called adaptability preparing on the grounds that it further develops adaptability. Adaptability preparation is intended to work on your versatility and scope of movement. While certain individuals decide to extend all alone, it's generally expected suggested that you stretch with the assistance of an actual specialist or ensured coach who can help change your stretches depending on the situation to make them High-impact activities, for example, strolling, running, running, cycling and swimming are great decisions for seniors hoping to expand their

pulse and consume additional calories. These activities will likewise help

assemble perseverance and work on your respiratory framework so you
can inhale better when taking part in everyday exercises. In the event that you're simply making changes in your workout daily schedule, begin slow and step by step develop your endurance after some time.
A few seniors might need to incorporate strength-preparing practices into
their regular exercise schedule. Strength-preparing practices are intended to assist you with developing your muscles, which can expand your solidarity and assist you with keeping a sound weight. Assuming you're
searching for ways of working on your general well-being by adding muscle strength, pushups, and pull-ups can be an extraordinary method for getting everything rolling. These activities fortify the back, shoulders, and
arms and are kind to the joints by neutralizing gravity rather than opposite muscle compressions.

Chapter 1

The Significance of Practicing For Seniors

Many individuals who are more established than 60 years of age might have their well-being decline on the off chance that they don't work out. There are enormous advantages
to participating in weight-bearing activities, like working on bone thickness, reinforcing the heart and lungs, bringing down

circulatory strain and cholesterol levels, and dialing back mental degradation and the sky is the limit from there. Seniors will actually want to live for a more drawn-out time frame in the event that they practice since practicing won't just increment actual development however it will likewise help mental excitement.

Regardless of what your age is or the amount you've been doing since before your twenties, there's not a great explanation for why you ought to be rusty any longer. You can make it happen if you have any desire to feel better, get in shape, and carry on with a solid life.

What is Exercise ?

The most effective way to characterize practice is by saying that it's a physical

a movement that you perform to help keep up with or work on your

wellbeing. Strolling around your area or going for a stroll in

the recreation area are extraordinary ways of working out. Observe that pretty much nothing remains to be prevented you from practicing inside assuming you favor this wellness strategy over going outside. You don't need to leave your

way occasionally on the grounds that it's the colder time of year. You can walk

around the house, make short goes around the block, and do sit-ups in your room; the significant thing here is: moving your

body.

What is Weight-Bearing Activity?

Weight-bearing activities are those exercises that include the

bones and muscles that make up your muscles. These exercises
should be possible in a club, at home, or elsewhere where you can run
around, hop and bounce while performing proactive tasks like
running, hopping, or working out with a rope. Running on a treadmill may
not be pretty much as fun as a round of football with your companions, yet at the same, it's still
a significant piece of weight-bearing activity for grown-ups more than 60.
Practice is Perfect for Both Your Psychological and Actual Wellbeing
One of the manners in which exercise can help your emotional wellness is by
assisting you with adapting to pressure when you have it. For instance,
studies have shown that when seniors feel worried, partaking in a type of weight-bearing activity will assist them with bettering
handle the pressure than if they sit idle. So on the off chance that you're having an upsetting day, get out and take a run or stroll around the
block. At the point when you feel quite a bit improved in the wake of working out, it's more straightforward for your body to quit having such a lot of cortisol (the stress chemical).
Practice is likewise awesome for working on your state of mind. When your
body discharges endorphins in the cerebrum, you feel like you're high

despite the fact that no medications are involved. These blissful sentiments from
endorphins make you bound to be content and assist you with remaining
positive over the course of the day. So despite the fact that you will not consistently
feel like it, practice is critical to keep yourself solid and solid.
Since seniors are bound to put on weight, practice is even more significant for them than for more youthful individuals. By taking part in weight-bearing activities, you can assist yourself with being better and more grounded. You won't stress over having issues
doing customary things on the grounds that your muscles will have areas of strength to be adequately adaptable to do anything that you want to do whenever.
You can't totally try not to put on weight as you age.
All things considered, by practicing routinely and being solid, you will not have an
issue with it getting really awful.
As you progress in years, the body loses bulk and deftness. By partaking in weight-bearing activities, you can work on those
things and assist your body with being really solid. A portion of the
benefits that come from practicing include:
• Assists with forestalling osteoporosis
• Assists with diminishing back torment
• Assists with expanding bone thickness
• Works on cardiovascular wellness
• Decreases feelings of anxiety
Practicing is extremely critical to carry on with a long

furthermore, solid life. Assume you need to be dynamic and partake

in proactive tasks as a grown-up. All things considered, you need to engage in weight-bearing activity. In time, you will not generally dislike your muscles in light of the fact that they'll be solid and adaptable enough to do all that you really want. Many individuals have the confusion that practicing is a task they should do. This issue can keep going for years, even many years. In

this part, I will give tips to assist you with fostering the propensity for

figuring out in any event, when you would rather not do it at this moment. These

tips have assisted me with turning out to be more focused and propelled to

work out.

1. Never skirt an exercise.

This is the most troublesome recommendation on the rundown to follow; all things considered, the issue is getting into the attitude to work out. Yet, listen to this: you can't get into an exercise mentality without working

out. Fortunately, as you make work-out schedules.

Plan two to four exercises each week and stick to them. Will be there in no time flat

days when you don't want to resolve, yet except if you're debilitated,

compel yourself to do as such. You can stop your exercise or do

something basic. Making wellness a propensity is critical to have a functioning life. It'll be significantly simpler to adhere to a routine after that.

2. Find something you appreciate doing.

You won't make some decent memories in the event that you scorn running but force yourself onto the treadmill. Finding an action you appreciate
is the way to get into the proper attitude.
Running, circular use, cycling, studio courses, and different choices are accessible. Working out at home will turn out to be a lot
simpler once you have a most loved action.
3. Lay out objectives and keep a visual record of your advancement.
In the event that you don't feel like you're gaining any headway, you could find
it challenging to rouse yourself to work out. No one appreciates working for no compensation, however, you may be gaining more headway than you
understand. Putting forth characterized objectives and keeping tabs on your development over
time is the best technique to conquer this issue.
For instance, each treadmill run might feel something very similar, however, if you
track your exercises, you might see that your speed has developed or
that you can run for longer periods. Various applications are accessible
to assist you with following your exercises, or you might utilize a standard scratch pad. Furthermore, accept me when I say that advancement is
fulfilling and will make them return for more!
4. Search for motivation
Words usually can't do a picture justice and may likewise expand your
inspiration by 1,000 percent. So encircle yourself with pictures

that rouse you to be dynamic assuming you want that additional push to
go to exercise at home. This could be a picture of your top most
competitor, others' advancement, or photographs of a fantasy area
like Mount Everest.
You can add a portion of visual inspiration to your day by making a
Interest notice board, following your top most competitors on Instagram,
or on the other hand removing photos from wellness magazines. Your way of life change will be directed by this vision board.
5. Remind yourself why you're carrying on with a functioning life Each time you work out, remind yourself why you joined the
club in any case. Consider how blissful you'll be at the point at which you
accomplish your targets. You're effective financial planning time and work that will
pay off later, and it will be in every way advantageous.
Regardless of whether working out seems a disturbance, embracing a thankful
outlook and valuing your body's capacity to move might make
each sweat meeting more agreeable. Get to work!

Chapter 2

How Seniors Can Begin

In the event that you are keen on beginning an exercise plan but have falterings or don't have the foggiest idea where to begin, there could be no greater time than

presently. A large portion of your retirement years will be spent in the solace of

your home, and you can utilize that chance to get fit and sound!

Begin with essential developments like squats, push-ups, sit-ups, and

lurches. Then, you'll tone muscles and take actions like getting

up from a situated position more straightforwardly and helping your equilibrium.

However, make a point not to exhaust yourself! Just set the objective for 5

more minutes of activity every day until you're as long as 30 minutes.

Restricted versatility or actual limitations might make certain

kinds of activity imprudent. Have an in depth discussion with your Doctor about the best practices for you. Begin gradually to stay away from injury and increment how much time spent being physical as you feel better. Make it a point to your primary care physician in the event that you have various forms of feedback.

Oxygen-consuming activities are any movement that utilizes enormous muscle gatherings,

which expands your heart siphoning and breath rate. Low-effect practices like strolling, swimming, and cycling are perfect
decisions that adversely influence the joints.
The NIA suggests 15O minutes seven days of moderate oxygen consuming
movement or 75 minutes per seven-day stretch of fiery high-impact workout, or
the comparable mix of moderate and enthusiastic movement.
Your exercise ought to be shifted and utilize every one of the muscles in your
body. On the off chance that you're simply beginning, center around building your perseverance prior to endeavoring further developed practices like running and swimming.
Center around lessening pressure however much as could reasonably be expected while doing any
active work. Stress increments cortisol in our bodies, driving
to loss of bulk and capability, low energy levels, lower digestion, and weight gain.
Attempt to clear your brain and dispose of every feeling of apprehension. Do this by paying attention to music or other calming sounds yet stay away from upsetting TV programs and discussions with requesting
individuals.
Notwithstanding stress decrease, yoga and reflection have been
displayed to have a few other medical advantages, including getting to the next level
lung limit, more grounded insusceptible framework, and better relaxing.

Certain individuals feel overpowered by the possibility of beginning a new

exercise routine daily practice so considers a novice's wellness class for your most memorable endeavor at a workout.

The initial step is significant on the grounds that disappointment assists you with the understanding

that you can fulfil what you set your heart to do. Then, at that point, you'll take

that data and apply it to different exercises.

Begin with something straightforward like strolling for a couple of moments a

day. Tracking your advancement will go far toward

persuading you to stay with actual work all through your

life. You can monitor your advancement by wellness journaling,

which is recording your exercise information, as well as the reasons

why you practiced and how they affected you.

Recollect that there is nobody size-fits-all exercise program.

Attempt various activities, find ones that are ideal for yourself, and make

sure the routine is charming!

Chapter 3

Step-by-step instructions to Move toward the Exercise

The advantages of heating up are amazing. As a matter of fact, it's no misrepresentation to say that heating up is one of the keys to partaking in a
solid life.
Heating up can assist you with forestalling muscle wounds, assuaging joint
torment, and keep up with execution all through your exercises. In the event that
you're not cautious, be that as it may, heart-capturing conditions, for example,
respiratory failure or stroke are bound to occur on the off chance that you don't warm up appropriately.
Your body's course framework isn't working as expected when
you're cold. However, on the off chance that you start with a decent warm-up, you'll get the flow moving, and it will keep on working appropriately over the course of your day.
At the point when you do a warm-up practice accurately, every joint, muscle
gathering, and organ benefits from the interaction. This sets the stage
for your whole day's exercise to be useful and agreeable.
For instance, toward the beginning of the day, I typically do running for around 20

minutes on the treadmill before I leave bed at 8:30 am. This

is one illustration of how a warm-up can assist me with performing better over the course of the day. I feel solid and certain realizing that I got my blood streaming prior to confronting my other exercises,

which can be very requested.

Then again, on the off chance that you don't heat up as expected, your exercise

can without much of a stretch become a disaster and a total misuse of your time.

The fat-consuming impacts of an activity meeting will diminish,

alongside strength-building power. That's another disadvantage

you're more well-suited to encounter muscle injury or joint agony at

some point.

Chapter 4

Dynamic Stretches and Static Stretches

In the realm of sports, dynamic stretches are turning out to be more

furthermore, more famous contrasted with static extending. It's a typical

misinterpretation that static extending is better for heating up.

in any case, truly: dynamic stretches have such countless advantages
over static stretches that it's no big surprise they're moving.
In this part, we'll be talking about why you ought to pick dynamic
extends over static stretches for heating up.

The Advantages of Dynamic Extending
There are a couple of explicit advantages that unique extending has
over static extending. At the point when a muscle is heated up, it can get
solid and difficult to move. At the point when this occurs, static extending will
assist with relaxing the muscle and make it more flexible. Notwithstanding,
there are numerous disadvantages to static extending for heating up.
Static stretches can be monotonous in light of the fact that you should continue to change points and positions all through the daily schedule. Not exclusively is this
counterproductive, yet it can actually hurt.
Dynamic extending can significantly diminish the time it takes to
warm up muscles. Your muscles will be tenderly extended all things considered
of being held under outrageous pressure by zeroing in on moving at the right point and position.
This permits your muscles to unwind, bringing about upgraded execution and less injury. It additionally implies greater adaptability all through
your exercise.

There are several advantages dynamic extending has while working out that static extending doesn't give. To begin, dynamic

stretches will assist with easing firmness and irritation that frequently feel

after an exercise meeting. The speedy development of dynamic

stretches will assist with expanding blood dissemination, which will bring

new oxygen and supplements to your muscles.

Your body will recuperate quicker and all the more proficiently after each

meeting. Dynamic extending additionally further develops coordination,

equilibrium, and attention to your body position. Along these lines, your

exercises will be more successful and productive. In the line of events you aspiring to further develop execution in your home or on the field at work, then

dynamic extending is an unquestionable necessity!

As you can see from this part, dynamic stretches have a lot of

benefits over static extending. By utilizing dynamic stretches before static stretches, you can support your body's exhibition in

your home while additionally disposing of any firmness you might have.

Assume you need to acquire better adaptability, work on joint versatility, or simply have a strong exercise. All things considered, I ask you to check dynamic loosening up!

Dynamic Stretches

Dynamic stretches are extending practices that move a joint through the entire accessible scope of movement or full length, yet no farther than that reach. Dynamic extending is a sort of stretch that includes moving pieces of your body and continuously expanding reach, speed of development, or both. The point of dynamic extending is to set up your body for practice by initiating the sensory system and raising the pulse. To guarantee that your dynamic stretches are protected and successful and keep away from injury, we suggest that you don't propel yourself excessively hard or quickly.

Dynamic stretches ought to be finished toward the start of an activity meeting to plan muscles for action as well as increment the scope of movement. Dynamic extending is helpful to competitors and dynamic individuals since it builds blood and oxygen stream and plans muscles for actual work. Dynamic extending additionally offers numerous different advantages, for example,

• Helped muscle coordination and capability
• Created nimbleness and adaptability
• Better equilibrium
• Worked on athletic execution

Dynamic Stretch Models

Hip Circles

• Stand on one leg, contacting a wall or seat for help if fundamental.
• Arch the foot on your other leg, delicately swinging your leg around in little circles.
• Perform 20 circles prior to exchanging legs.
• Stir up to bigger circles as your adaptability creates.

Shoulder Circles

• Stand with your feet shoulder-width separated and lift your arms out directly to the side at shoulder level.

• Begin making little circles with your hands and step by step increment the size, stirring up to bigger circles. Perform 20 circles.

• Turn around the course of your circles and rehash.

What Are Static Stretches?

Static stretches are delicate stretches that you hold for a while, and accompany many advantages. The point of a static stretch is to move your muscles to the extent that they can do without feeling any aggravation, then, at that point, stand firm on that foothold for 20-30 seconds. Rehash the stretch 2-3 times each time you perform it. To keep your stretches protected and viable, recollect: begin gradually, don't extend past what's agreeable, be delicate with your developments, and make sure to relax!

Static stretches can be utilized previously or after an exercise, however, research demonstrates the way that static extending before an exercise can really accompany a few expected gambles. In a perfect world, static stretches ought to be performed after your exercise to receive the rewards. This is on the grounds that static extending affects the muscles and the body, which might actually impede athletic execution whenever utilized before an exercise. This isn't to imply that static extending ought to never be utilized pre-exercise, yet do so sparingly.

Despite this, static stretches accompany many advantages, including:

• Further developed development productivity and adaptability

• Better unwinding

• Diminishes muscle pressure and touchiness

• Brings down the gamble of lower back torment

Static Stretch Models

Hamstring Stretch

• Sit with the two legs stretched out straight.
• While pivoting at the midsection, broaden your arms and reach forward similarly as feels great. Try to keep your knees straight.
• Hold for 20 to 30 seconds.
• Discharge once more into the beginning position.
• Rehash multiple times.
Quad Stretch
• Stand with the two feet together so your knees are contacting.
• Shift your weight onto one foot and lift the impact point of the other. Contact the wall or a seat in the event that you want additional soundness.
• Handle the rear of the lifted foot utilizing the hand on a similar side, and pull it in towards your glutes. Push your hips in a forward direction and chest cranial.
• Stand firm on the footing for 20 to 30 seconds, then switch legs and rehash.

Chapter 5

Heating/ Warm Up Activities

Permit 5 to 10 minutes for your pre-practice warm-up (or somewhat longer in a chilly climate).
On the off chance that you are practicing at a more significant level than for general wellness, or have a specific brandishing objective as a primary concern, you might require a more extended warm-up, and one that is planned explicitly for your game.
Warm-up choices

Follow these choices in the request recorded.

1. General warm-up

To start your warm-up complete 5 minutes of light (low force) actual work like strolling, running on the spot or on a trampoline, or cycling. Siphon your arms or make enormous however controlled roundabout developments with your arms to assist with warming the muscles of your chest area.

2. Sport-explicit warm-up

One of the most incredible ways of heating up is to play out the impending activity at a sluggish speed. This will permit you to reenact at low force the developments you are going to perform at higher power during your picked action. Common models incorporate consistent running, cycling, or swimming previously

advancing to a quicker speed. This may then be trailed by a few game explicit developments and exercises, for example, a couple of moments of simple getting practice for cricketers or baseball players, going through the movement of bowling a ball for grass bowlers, shoulder rolls or evading and slow-paced practice hits for tennis players. Sport-explicit warm-ups are many times planned by a certified coach in that game.

3. Extending

Any extending is best performed after your muscles are warm, so just stretch after your general warm-up. Extending muscles when they are cold and less flexible may prompt a tear. Extending during a warm-up can incorporate some sluggish, controlled circumnavigating developments at key joints, for example, shoulder rolls, yet the stretches ought not to be constrained or done at a speed that might extend the joint, muscles, and ligaments past their typical length.

One more part of extending during a warm-up is 'static extending' — where a muscle is tenderly extended and stood firm on the extended foothold for 10-30 seconds. This is by and large thought to be the most secure technique for extending.

Play out a light static extending routine toward the finish of your warm-up by extending every one of the muscle bunches you will use in your picked movement. A static stretch ought to be held where you can feel the stretch but experience no inconvenience. In the event that you feel uneasiness, move back on the stretch. Recall not to bob while holding the stretch.

Concentrates on looking at a warm-up that incorporates static extending with a warm-up that does exclude static extending have shown that pre-practice static extending further develops adaptability, however, its impact on injury counteraction stays indistinct. Subsequently, you might find it better to keep the vast majority of your static extending for after your activity meeting, or at least, as a feature of your cool-down.

Aside from static extending, different techniques for extending incorporate ballistic, dynamic, and PNF (proprioceptive neuromuscular help) extending, every one of which is best finished under guidance from a certified health specialist or sports mentor.

Chapter 6

10mins work out

How about we get to the quick and dirty and hop into this full-body exercise that scratches off the appropriate boxes? This full-body exercise could get the job done as it's just 10 minutes in length and will make them train your whole body as far as possible.

This exercise is quite serious, so if you're in a rush and need to get your heart siphoning, it's the full-body exercise for you. We suggest perusing the bearings for each activity (see beneath) to ensure that you comprehend how to execute every one preceding the beginning of the exercise. Whenever you have an outline, now is the ideal time to begin — get out your stopwatch and get going! You'll complete two rounds of the accompanying:

• Bouncing jacks — 1 moment
• Push-ups (normal or against a wall) — 30 seconds
• Hip-ups — 30 seconds on each side (left/right)
• Shudder kicks — 30 seconds
• Single leg glute spans — 30 seconds on each side (left/right)
• Wall sits — 1 moment

Hopping jacks

Muscles included: Calves, quads, glutes, upper back

Bearings:

• Stand with your feet closed and your arms tight at your sides.

• In one movement, bounce your feet out to each side and raise your arms over your head.

• Promptly converse the movement to get back to the beginning position.

Tips:

• Keep your arms directly consistently

• Remain light on feet and bounce as discreetly as could be expected

Customary push-ups

Muscles included: Chest, shoulders, rear arm muscles, upper back, abs

In the event that you can't finish push-ups with appropriate structure look at the wall variety down beneath! Put your hands level on the ground, straightforwardly under your shoulders with your feet somewhat more extensive than hip-width separated on the floor.

Headings:

• Step your legs out straight behind you with your feet together and toes twisted under.

• Tense each muscle to shape a straight line from your head through to your heels.

• Then, bring down your chest to the ground, keeping your elbows tight to your body.

• Expand your arms, then drive your body away from the beginning back to the beginning position.

Tips:

• Keep your neck in accordance with your spine with your shoulders back and away from your ears

• To diminish trouble: put your hands on a higher surface

• To increment trouble: put feet on a higher surface

Wall push-ups

Muscles included: Chest, shoulders, rear arm muscles, upper back, abs

These are the ideal transformation in the event that you don't yet have the solidarity to finish customary push-ups with great structure. Excessively simple? Then, at that point, do your push-ups on a surface at hip level, for example, put your hands on a table for help.

Bearings:

• Put your hands on a wall at chest level, and keep your wrists in accordance with your shoulders.

• Tense your muscles to frame a straight line from your head through to your heels.

• Then, bring down your chest to the wall, keeping your elbows tight to your body.

• Switch the development and push your body away from the wall, then, at that point, lower back to the beginning position.

Tips:

• Keep your neck long with shoulders back and down away from ears

• Draw in the center all through

Hip-ups

Muscles included: Abs, shoulders

Bearings:

• Lie on your side with your lower arm on the floor and elbows straightforwardly under your shoulders with your hips and feet stacked.

• Raise your hips off the floor, so your body frames a straight line from your head through to your heels.

• Lift your hips as high as conceivable while keeping them stacked.

• Gradually further your hips down to the beginning position.

Tips:

• Keep your neck stretch out with your shoulders caudal and down away from your ears

Ripple Kicks

Muscles included: Abs, lower back, quads
Headings:
• Lie on your back with your hands under your hips, your lower back ought to be squeezed into the floor and your legs raised a few crawls off the ground.
• With your legs straight all through, move one advantage and one leg down.
• Invert the development of your legs to make a light shudder development.
Tips:
• Keep your back squeezed into the floor consistently
Single-leg Glute Scaffolds
Muscles included: Glutes, hamstrings, abs
Headings:
• Lie on your back with your knees bowed and your feet level on the floor.
• Lift one leg directly to frame a 45° point to the floor.
• Drive your weight into the impact point of the foot on the floor and raise your hips to shape a straight line from shoulders through to your knees and toes.
• Stop at the highest point of the development, connect with your center, and agreement your glutes.
• Lower your hips back down to the beginning position.
Tips:
• Fasten your shoulders back and down, away from your ears
• Keep your hips squared — one hip bone ought to never be higher than the other
Wall Sits
Muscles included: Hamstrings, quads, glutes, abs
Bearings:
• Stand with your whole back and heels contacting the wall.

• Step the two feet one and a half feet forward while keeping your back squeezed into the wall.
• Without much space to move, continuously lower yourself until your legs are bowed at a 90°angle as though letting down to sit in a seat.
• Stand firm on this foothold for the assigned time.
Tips:
• Keep your body in an orderly fashion and your hands off your thighs

Chapter 7

THE COOL-DOWN

Why cool down?
The act of chilling off after practice implies dialing back your degree of movement steadily.
Chilling off:
• helps your pulse and breathing to return to resting levels continuously;
• abstains from swooning or unsteadiness, which can result from blood pooling in the enormous muscles of the legs when energetic movement is halted out of nowhere;
• assists with eliminating metabolites (middle substances shaped during digestion) from your muscles, for example, lactic corrosive, which can develop during lively action (lactic corrosive is most successfully taken out by delicate activity as opposed to halting abruptly); and
• readies your muscles for the following activity meeting, whether it's the following day or in a couple of days' time.

You might see clashing exhortation regarding whether chilling off forestalls post-practice muscle irritation, otherwise called deferred beginning muscle touchiness (DOMS), which will in general happen in the wake of doing the new activity or working at a harder level than expected. In any case, regardless of whether chilling off forestall DOMS, different advantages of chilling off imply that you ought to constantly make it a piece of your activity meeting.

DOMS is more normal after new activity including 'flighty' muscle constrictions, like running downhill, or bringing downloads, as the muscles are placed under more pressure than typical in these exercises. Be that as it may, such irritation typically just happens in the initial not many meetings, since the muscles adjust, and with kept preparing shouldn't happen.

Guaranteeing a compelling cool-down

For a compelling cool-down:

• perform low-power practice for at least 5 to 10 minutes; and

• follow this with an extended schedule.

Cool-down choices

1. Proceeding with your picked practice while steadily bringing down its power

Step-by-step dialing back the speed and effort of your movement for more than a few minutes can appear to be a characteristic movement, as well as satisfying the need to incorporate a cool-down period toward the finish of your activity.

2. Slow running, energetic strolling, or delicate cycling

Another choice is to run, walk energetically, or cycle for a couple of moments after your activity, ensuring that this action is lower in power than the activity you have recently performed.

Extending as a feature of your cool-down

The best chance to extend is during your cool-down, as right now your muscles are still warm and probably going to answer well, and there is an okay of injury. Extending assists with loosening up your muscles and reestablishing them to their resting length, and further developing adaptability (the scope of development about your joints).

As a guide, permit 10 minutes of post-practice extending for each hour of activity. Make these post-practice extends more intensive than your pre-practice extends. Guarantee that you stretch all the significant muscle bunches that you have utilized during your activity. Stretch each muscle bunch for 20 to 30 seconds, 2 to multiple times.

Chapter 8

Remaining sound late in the game

Regardless of your age, it's critical to deal with your body and forestall sickness.

Be that as it may, in the event that you're 65 or more established, something as straightforward as this season's virus or a typical virus can advance and prompt entanglements. This incorporates optional diseases like pneumonia, bronchitis, ear contamination, or a sinus disease. In the event that you have a persistent condition, for example, asthma or diabetes, a respiratory disease can exacerbate these.

Along these lines, it means a lot to pursue solid decisions to reinforce your invulnerable framework and decrease the probability of sickness.

Follow these nine hints to remain sound all year.

1. Get dynamic

Actual work is a safe framework sponsor. The more you are mobile. the more your body can tackle aggravation and infirmities.

The action you participate in doesn't need to be exhausting. Low-effect practices are viable, as well.

You should seriously mull over trekking, strolling, swimming, or low effect heart stimulating exercise. In the event that you're ready to, take part in moderate power practice for around 20 to 30 minutes per day to arrive at the suggested all out of 150 minutes a weekTrusted Source. Likewise, reinforce your muscles by lifting loads or doing yoga.

After your workout daily practice find what feels best for you.

2. Accept supplements as the need should arise

A few enhancements assist with supporting a solid resistant framework. Prior to taking an enhancement, consistently inquire as to whether it's protected, particularly on the off chance that you're taking a professionally prescribed medicine. A few enhancements they might suggest incorporate calcium, vitamin D, vitamin B6, or vitamin B12.

Accept enhancements or multivitamins as educated to support your safe framework.

3. Eat a sound eating regimen

Consuming fewer calories wealthy in organic products, vegetables, and lean meats likewise gives your safe framework a lift and safeguard against destructive infections and microorganisms that cause diseases. Foods grown from the soil are a wonderful wellspring of cell reinforcements. Cancer prevention agents safeguard your cells from harm and keep your body sound.

You ought as far as possible your utilization of sweet and greasy food sources, which can set off irritation in the body and lower your safe framework.

Likewise, limit your admission of liquor. Get quality ideas concerning safety measures of liquor to drink per day or week.

4. Clean up every now and again

Cleaning up consistently is one more magnificent method for remaining sound all year. Infections can survive on surfaces for as long as a whole day. It's feasible to turn out to be sick in the event that you contact with an infection-covered surface and defile your hands, and contact your face.

Clean up with warm lathery water frequently, and for no less than 20 seconds. Try not to contact your nose, face, and mouth with your hands.

You can likewise safeguard yourself by utilizing antibacterial hand sanitizer when you can't clean up. Additionally, clean surfaces around your home and workstation oftentimes.

5. Figure out how to oversee pressure

Persistent pressure expands your body's creation of the pressure chemical cortisol. An excess of cortisol can upset various capabilities in your body, including your safe framework.

To diminish pressure, increment actual work, get a lot of rest, set sensible assumptions for yourself, and investigate unwinding, charming exercises.

6. Get a lot of rest

In addition to the fact that rest lessens can your anxiety, rest is the means by which your body fixes itself. Hence, getting a sufficient measure of rest can bring about a more grounded invulnerable framework, making it simpler for your body to ward off infections.

Rest is additionally significant as you progress in years since it can further develop memory and fixation. Hold back nothing seven and a half to nine hours of rest each evening.

Assuming you experience difficulty dozing, converse with your primary care physician to track down the fundamental reason. Reasons for a sleeping disorder can incorporate idleness during the day and a lot of caffeine. Or on the other hand, it very well may be an indication of an ailment like rest apnea or a propensity to fidget.

7. Do whatever it takes to forestall diseases

Getting yearly immunizations is one more method for remaining sound consistently. On the off chance that you're age 65 and more seasoned, converse with your PCP about getting a high-portion or adjuvant influenza immunization.

Influenza season is between October and May in the US. It requires around fourteen days for the immunization to be viable, and it lessens the gamble of influenza by 40 to 60 percent trusted Source when the antibody strains match the flowing strains.

The seasonal infection changes every year, so you ought to get the immunization yearly. You can likewise converse with your primary care physician about getting pneumococcal immunizations to safeguard against pneumonia and meningitis.

8. Plan yearly physicals

Booking a yearly exam can likewise keep you solid. Continuously talk with your PCP assuming you have worries about your well-being.

Conditions like diabetes and hypertension can go undetected. Standard actual assessments will empower your primary care physician to early analyze any issues. Seeking early treatment might forestall long-haul complexities.

Likewise, assuming you have any cold or influenza side effects, see your PCP right away. The seasonal infection can prompt confusion in grown-ups beyond 65 years old. The safe framework debilitates with age, making it harder to ward off the infection.

In the event that you see a specialist within the initial 48 hours of influenza side effects, they can recommend an antiviral to diminish the seriousness and length of side effects.

9. Keep away from contact with individuals who are wiped out

One more method for safeguarding yourself all year is to try not to be near individuals who are wiped out. This is much tougher to do than one might expect. However, on the off chance that there's an influenza flare-up in your space, limit contact with individuals who aren't feeling good and keep away from swarmed regions until conditions get to the next level.

On the off chance that you should go out, safeguard yourself by wearing a facial covering. In the event that you're really focusing on somebody with this season's virus, wear a facial covering and gloves, and clean up often.

Conclusion

Advancing with age is a very beautiful, one to be enjoyed as much as possibly. Regardless, there could be a lot of obstacles to living your advanced years in vitality and vigor. This book has been carefully put together to help seniors get around with spring in their feet as in their youthful age.   What to and what not to do has been complied for your good. Stay back, relax and embrace being a senior.